GW00859560

WASP DISENTANGLEMEN

Gordon Vells works as a translator and editor from his home, close to the point where the counties of Dorset, Somerset and Wiltshire meet.

Wasp Disentanglement for Beginners is the sequel to his first poetry collection, *Plundered by Lobsters*.

Gordon Vells is a pen-name.

More poetry by Gordon Vells in Xenon Lobster Books:

Plundered by Lobsters

On Wings

Wasp Disentanglement *for* Beginners

Poems of nature, landscape and memory

Gordon Vells

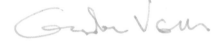

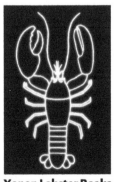

Xenon Lobster Books

First published in 2022 by Xenon Lobster Books

ISBN 978-1-4717-3847-0

Typeset in Constantia

Printed by Lulu.com

Xenon Lobster Books
1 Pimpernel Court, Gillingham,
Dorset SP8 4UW, England

www.xenonlobster.co.uk
@xenonlobster

For Dad.

I know you liked the one about the cloud chamber.

Contents

Wasp Disentanglement for Beginners

Should you ever encounter
a wasp entangled in a cobweb
and feel compelled
to release it,
you would do well
to remember this:
no wasp has ever demonstrated gratitude,
other than by stinging.

About the diagrams:

I wanted to find a way to convey the variation in size of wasp species without scaring the life and breath out of my more squeamish readers. These diagrams, which are life-size, are my attempt to do that. They roughly illustrate the body size, wingspan and (in dotted lines) limb spread of each species.

If these symbolic representations are still too much for you, you can of course surgically remove those pages from the book, burn them and jump up and down on the ashes screaming until you feel better. I'll quite understand.

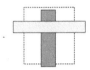

Vespula vulgaris

Length: 15 mm; wingspan: 20 mm

The common wasp. Sometimes annoyingly common. Where I grew up, in North Dorset, we always used to call them "jaspers". Maybe you still do.

Morning Walks One

Fifteen years ago I saw a kingfisher from this bridge.
Oh, the briefest of glimpses, sure –
but that split-second of blue and orange
has kept me coming back
and every day I pause and look in case.

Just the briefest of glimpses, this life:
a brilliant metallic flash, then gone.

First Aid

There are a pair of sticking-plasters on the pavement
crossed in the shape of an X.
They've been there for several weeks.
Perhaps some kind soul saw
that the tarmac was injured
and administered some caring first aid.
I'd like to know whether the pavement has healed yet,
but I don't want to remove the plasters
and destroy this tiny work of art.

Lannacombe

we stop,
stretch two souls on the sand;

a quicksilver brook bounces the sunlight around us
and empties into the green-white sea
that falls towards us without rest,

each wave a geological moment
infinitesimally shaping the black rocks
that frame the beach
and bound our being

Before Sunrise

pure, chaste snow
three thumbs thick or more

every step is intoxicating
I just want another

the feel of the crunch
the crumpling, crinkling squeak of the flakes compressing

sharper on tarmac, softer on grass
with an added crack if you break hidden ice beneath

this sound-dampened dawn
preternaturally still

except for the winter stream
and one magpie chiching

I'd forgotten this feeling
how snow halves my age

no, I will not take the shortcut home
I want more

Tree Hugger

On my way back from the shops
I saw a man clinging to a tree,
as if afraid that he or it would float away;
I didn't like to ask which.

Cloud Chamber

Between me and the sun,
water droplets and ideas dance in the air –
some swirl and shine;
others fade and sink.

Here I am in the mist,
in the midst of all this unexpected light,
waiting for muons
in my cloud chamber.

Tåkekammer

*Mellom meg og solen
danser vanndråper og idéer i luften –
noen virvler og glitrer;
andre svinner hen, synker ned.*

*Her er jeg i skodden,
omgitt av alt dette uventede lyset,
ventende på myoner
i mitt tåkekammer.*

Childhood Trauma

I have two scars from childhood,
both incurred around the age of four or five.
One is on my forehead
where I ran into a piano
in a blaze of excitement,
extinguished by blood and stitches;
the other, deeper scar
was left by the liver and baked beans
I was forced to eat at school –
the grim, metallic gristle
chewed cold and alone while others played –
and though the thought of those supposèd foods
still turns my stomach,
curiously, I love the piano more than ever,
bump on head notwithstanding.

Electrostephanus petiolatus

Length: 10 mm; wingspan: 10 mm

An extinct species of crown wasp known only from a single specimen preserved in Baltic amber.

Wasp Cartography

Your brittle body
is an ancient map:
continents, seas, islands
in orpiment and lampblack.

I trace the roadways
on your bitter wing,
every fork and junction
a reminder of choices made.

Rounding the headland,
a lighthouse, an eye;
unsafe harbours, mouthparts;
radio masts, antennae.

Fine hairs on thorax
like surveyor's hatching
for an incline or cutting:
cartographic projection.

Through the contours
of the insect landscape,
a sensory safari
to your peninsula of war.

Your little brittle corpse,
a few grams' heavy light –
the mapmaker's handiwork
in orpiment and lampblack.

Archaeology

The Velcro on your coat
is archaeology,
telling tales
of every jumper and scarf you've worn.

Trails

Snail trails at my feet
mirror the criss-crossing vapour trails above –
people in a hurry to get somewhere else.
Do snails feel like they're moving fast, I wonder,
in the same way that air travel's speed is almost
    imperceptible;
and do we ever really get to where we want to be?

Jazz Club

what music would you be making now
the year you turn eighty-four
if you were still

what music would we have made together
senior and junior
if I'd been any

what music is there left between us
I'll follow your chord progressions
let me sit in

The Viaduct

standing under the viaduct
with its echoes
every bee that passes a squadron
my thoughts resound as much as my voice

and those thoughts turn to you
of course they do
and they bounce off the brickwork
my soul echoing under the arches

Blue
(for Arabella)

Blue
is a cool hue:
glaciers are blue;
cold taps are labelled blue;
sub-zero temperatures on weather forecasts
    are always shown in blue.

So why is it, do you think,
that when we see blue skies above us,
it makes us feel warm inside?

The Gallery
(for Mum)

I first got to know this gallery
in half-height days.
Not unaccompanied, of course:
I had a personal curator and guide
who explained the meanings of the works.
Here a still life, glistening fruit piled;
there a collage,
an installation of school blazers and ties;
portraits of fish and meat;
bread in 4D scented oils;
dioramas of sweets and TVs.

When the years began with apostrophe-seven
there were pieces by artists
working in newsprint, toys and wool,
shoe happenings,
clockwork displays
and brightly coloured bottles.

Now the gallery is much changed.
Gone the masterpieces:
empty frames hang,
the canvases roughly hacked from their surrounds.
In place of missing works,
faded, peeling walls,
cobwebs,
nail holes,
five estate agents,
four charity shops
and a Costa Coffee.

Fizz-buzz

Age 12:
first German lesson.
The thrill of writing two little dots –
  fünf.
Hot on its heels,
the exhilarating swirsh and mystery –
  dreißig.

Age 29:
first Norwegian lesson.
Echoes of that childhood fizz of pen –
  sønn.
New shapes,
new pretzel tangles to master –
  lærer.

Age 50:
this page.
The joy there was in writing
  swirsh.
The buzz of writing
something you've never written before.

Burning Biros

The smell of burning Biro –
acrid tang of combusting plastic –
sticks a pin in time.

Chemistry classes:
potential for havoc caused by absence of teacher
combined with presence of Bunsen's finest invention.
Experiment 1: Determine the melting point of Bic pens;
draw out the softened barrel into a long, thin capillary tube;
inky smoke rises.

All this came back to me yesterday
as, biting into a ham sandwich, I found mustard:
the taste of burning Biro.

The Blackbird on Its High Branch Sings

the blackbird on its high branch sings
without repeating itself
a three-second composition
and then a pause for effect

the blackbird sings high in the tree
a new piece for three seconds
slightly different this time
after which an empty moment

silhouetted against the sky
blackbird song, three seconds long
non-repeating notes and trills
and now the earth breathes

on its high branch, the blackbird sings
never quite repeating
its three seconds of expression
and now I wait for the next one

Doing the Other Thing

Whenever it was
I don't precisely recall
but you said, apropos of something:
If they don't like it, they can just do the other thing –
determination,
mixed with a wordsome creativity
that sparkled with wit and vim,
and I loved that.

And now I reflect,
a decade since *I do*s,
that given the choice of two
predictable courses of action,
you'll do the other thing:
a creative third path that I hadn't foreseen,
sparkling with wit and vim,
and I love that.

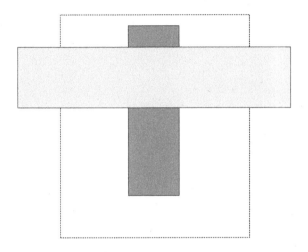

Vespa mandarinia

Length: 45 mm; wingspan: 75 mm

The Asian giant hornet is one of the world's largest wasps.
In North America it is often called the "murder hornet",
but in some parts of Japan the larvae are gathered
as a handy food source and the adults, once deep-fried,
are considered a tasty snack.

Hachinoko

crumbly   crunchy   creamy
    larval stage   baby wasp
                    entomophagous treat
        sugar on pupa
        c o m e   t o   t h e   e d i b l e   w a s p   f e s t i v a l
        eat and buy   canned   or pickled in sake
        first take your wasp larvae
    make   into   paste   with   soy   sauce   and   peanuts
                        spread onto sticky rice and grill
tasty for those too squeamish   squirmy   to eat them live
            rich in B vitamins
    the elderly villagers dig   their digger wasp crackers
                season to taste
    or deep-fry the adults   hachinoko
                            like granny made
            if feeling   really a d v e n t u r o u s
        try a salty giant hornet
                delicacy   so delicate
            without fearless
        u n l i m i t e d   c a p a c i t y   f o r   g r u b s

I Don't Like to Think about It

I don't like to think about it,
but I know the day will come.
How will I feel? Hard to know.
Sad for the loss, of course,
but the loss is so long past
I can hardly recall it.
Relieved that the struggle is over,
for your sake
and for ours;
guilty for feeling that;
annoyed about feeling guilty;
angry about feeling annoyed.

And what then?
There will be different concerns,
others to worry about –
there already are –
and I suppose
those anxieties will take over
as the firepot of emotions
gradually seethes more gently:
anger, guilt and grief replaced
by tender recollection,
reverberating absence,
and the nothing of being.

Then I'll go to the airfield
where so often you took me,
but this time alone,
and I'll watch the planes
as they escape the earth,
shrink,
fade,
and disappear into the past.

Vocation Vocation Vocation

If asked to state my occupation,
my default answer these days would be "Translator".
However, that's not something I do *every* day.
What I *do* do every day is bite myself.
Not really every child's dream, is it?

What do you want to do when you grow up, son?
I want to bite myself.
Do you now, lad?
Aye, Grandad, I do, it looks really exciting.

And indeed it is –
just when you think you're having a nice lunch
or just when you're admiring a colourful sunset
or just when you've fallen asleep
there it is:
c h o m p

You never know what's going to happen next in this game:
Will it be tongue, or cheek, or lip?
Will the shock make you yelp?
Will you draw blood?

Translation's a living;
poetry's a calling;
but biting yourself?
The career prospects are terrible,
but apparently my vocation's chosen *me*.

SD 080 906

the waves gently lullaby us
you slumber beside me
blue sky stretches from sea horizon
    to inland fellscape
with wisps and blobs of cloud as punctuation

this is the calmest I've felt in weeks
with the peace and the beauty
the sun warming my neck
and highlighting also in white
    the distant nuclear power station

Input

Please enter your real name in full.
By "real name in full" we mean
first name in the "first name" box
and surname in the "surname" box.
If your name doesn't neatly fit
into the strict boxes provided –
because you have three first names
or two surnames
or no surname
or your surname comes first –
that's just not good enough;
your real name is not acceptable
and you will have to change it
to suit our system.

Please enter your real name in full.
If you do not know your real name,
please enter your real name in full.
If you do not have a real name,
please enter it anyway,
because without your real name
we aren't interested.
If you cannot enter your name
because you cannot read or write
please enter your real name in full.

If to write your name
requires letters or characters not available on this system
or you cannot write your name
because it is in a language that has no written form
please enter your real name in full
using only the letters A to Z.
Nothing else is acceptable
and therefore your real name cannot include
any other characters.
Other alphabets or writing systems cannot be accepted.
Accents, apostrophes or hyphens cannot be accepted.
Your real name is what we say it is.
You will be assimilated.

What is your real name anyway?
Is it the name your parents gave you
when you were born
or even before you were born?
Is it the name you took
when you promised yourself to another?
Is it your sign name?
Is it the name your boss calls you?
Is it the name your family now call you?
Is it the name you have chosen for yourself?
Or is it the name that the system has forced upon you?

Choose carefully.

The Personality of Rain
(for Boof)

looking out this café window
at the sort of drizzle that doesn't so much fall as levitate
soaking pedestrians by stealth
I recall that a good friend once asked me
whether I felt that rain had more personality than sunshine
maybe there's something to that
this stuff is devious

one day on, and the rain is determined
a constant percussion like a hundred fingernails tapping on
    the car roof and windscreen
this rain is going nowhere, and it's got a job to do:
to wet-hit every blade of grass
every bump of tarmac
every knot of children
every coat and hat
to work its way in between every crack in every fence
down every collar
into every aching joint
determination in droplet form

the next day:
the rain is falling like angry nails
furiously drilling into anything in its path
a liquid assault on every sense
and now it's stopped
as suddenly as it started
like a child's tantrum
that could only be sustained for so long
another new personality

and I'll freely admit
that sometimes a shower can be refreshing
darkening the baked, dusty ground of summer
or a thunderstorm can bring relief
from oppressive, headachy skies
but today
after six straight hours of supercharged mist
punctuated only by heavier downpours
call me predictable
but right now
I'd settle for the benign personality vacuum of warm
    sunshine

Blastophaga psenes

Length: 2 mm; wingspan: 3.8 mm

One of the hundreds of species of wasps that pollinate figs.
If you like eating figs, reading up on fig wasps may not be
the best idea.

47

Seven Bowls: Fragments of Earth

I.

stumbling through
the burning forest
of all humanity's promises

II.

earthly remains:
sculptures of vultures
engravings of ravens
ozalids of chrysalids
photostats of meerkats
mimeographed giraffes
polystyrene thylacines
xeroxed aurochs
stuffed choughs
balloon raccoons
soon all that will be left
is lifeless, deathless replicas
simulacra
unsouls

III.

mankind
sold his kidney to buy an iPhone
sold his ears to get guilt-cancelling headphones
sold his planet to make shiny stuff that soon broke

IV.

the fourth angel poured out his bowl upon the sun
and power was granted to it to scorch mankind –
the species that burnt its own hat
and then complained of sunstroke –
and they repented not

V.

in a world
of emergency fixes
like a teetering pile of sticking-plasters
patching up a decapitation
or a tree
hollow, rotten and brittle
bound together by a pretty ribbon
but awaiting collapse

VI.

driving into the night
we can't see where we're going
retina-burning lights from every direction
not illuminating
just preventing sight
the drivers are blind and blissfully unaware
the passengers are screaming
cul-de-sac

VII.

the sky tonight
was the colour of tigers –
what have we done?

Fresh Air

I should open the windows for fresh air.

I will open the windows back and front,
and the through draught will scatter

all my papers
and all the dust.

Putting everything back the way it was
will give me something to do.

Perhaps I will open the windows.

You've Got a Lot to Answer for, Sigmund

You've got to have a dream,
apparently.
But I dispute that.
I'd be more than happy to be without dreams.

Dreams are a place where nothing makes sense,
where nothing connects,
where space and time are Möbius-shaped,
where long-dead friends meet impossible colleagues,
where I still have to go to school in my fifties,
where I can swim,
and fly,
and then wake up disappointed.

I could do without the distress of public underwear-based
    embarrassment,
being unable to outrun ants,
watching my car being crushed,
being shot,
getting into a punch-up with a famous journalist,
being unwillingly seduced by a many-headed gorgon,
being deceived by a friendly chap who turns out to be an
    evil lizard,
being shot again . . .

I *don't* got to have a dream.
Why would I want to experience any of this?
Dreams can come true, they say.
I certainly hope not.

Flutes

If you don't want to talk right now
that's fine, honest.
I'll just leave my ears on the side here,
a pair of flutes awaiting
whatever bottle you choose to uncork and pour.

The Young Road
(for Reidar)

We were young once,
piloting your battered, one-eyed Peugeot
through the northern tundra,
slowing for reindeer,
paddling in Arctic seas
and chasing the sun to North Cape.

We were young once,
braving the blizzards day and night,
driving – and sliding – on packed ice,
cursing army headlights,
running out of road in an island field
and laughing like drains.

We were young once,
following our noses to the ends of the roads,
all to the coolest soundtracks –
"Rock 'n' roll, Disco Duck."
Well, we still have more road trips in us;
we are still young.

Reality Judder

sitting, as I was,
in free air –
sun on face,
surrounded by the swirl of humanity,
the modern world in full effect,
all was well –
I momentarily glimpsed in my peripheral vision
that in their cross-sliding movement
      the clouds briefly stuttered
            reality juddered
and in that moment the illusion was broken

Sorting Options

The moons of Jupiter sorted alphabetically.
The moons of Jupiter sorted by size.
The moons of Jupiter sorted by roundness.
The moons of Jupiter sorted by year of discovery.
The moons of Jupiter sorted by odour.
The moons of Jupiter sorted by magnitude.
The moons of Jupiter sorted by pinkness.
The moons of Jupiter sorted by orbital eccentricity.
The moons of Jupiter sorted by my eccentricity.
The moons of Jupiter sorted by cuteness.
The moons of Jupiter sorted by resemblance to a badger.
The moons of Jupiter sorted by their names' resemblance
    to the word "badger".
The moons of Jupiter sorted randomly.
The moons of Jupiter sorted by name –
    not the names humans have given them,
    but the names Jupiter calls them.

Gratitude

Thank you, throbbing small-hours headache.
Without you,
I would not have abandoned hope of further sleep.
Without you,
I would not have witnessed the burnished dawn.
Without you,
I would not have ventured into the cool 5 a.m. air.
Without you,
I would not have seen
    the incredible light on the trees and the fields,
    caressed by the damp, post-shower sun.
Without you,
I would not have heard the song thrush
    composing and performing the greatest
    avant-garde concerto of the 21st century.
Without you,
throbbing small-hours headache,
I would not have embarked on this day
    in such a positive, creative frame of mind.

(promises)

I promise to be careful.
I promise I will always remain calm.
I promise not to give up.
I promise I don't snore.
I promise it wasn't me, as far as I can remember.
I promise I am sorry.
I promise love.
I promise tea.
I promise chocolate.
I promise to bring back glass from the moon.
I promise you giant moles wearing ludicrous hats.
I promise to keep my distance.
I promise to hold your hand.
I promise I will never.
I promise I will always.
I promise not to keep my promises, especially this one.

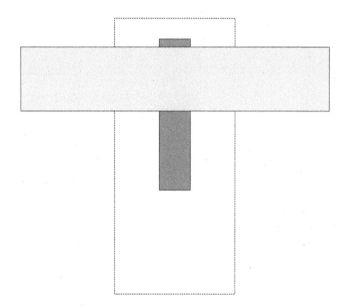

Pepsis grossa

Length: 40 mm; wingspan: 85 mm

A very large species of tarantula hawk wasp that,
as the name suggests, preys on big, furry spiders.
Its sting is reportedly among the most painful of all insects',
and the effect has been described as like being tasered.

Visiting Time

Can't even see your face.
All there is
is a shape of you,
a question mark of human
under hospital blanket.
Breathing-moving,
two three,
a little mouse exhalation,
two three,
every few counts.
It's hard to equate
this punctuation mark
with the person I knew.
Visiting time is over;
you haven't stirred.
Same as before
and before that.
Maybe you'll be awake tomorrow.

In These Days

in these days of grey and cloud
        someone broke the phoenix' neck
no fiery rebirth – not this time
        there will be no reconnect

the line's been cut and all our calls
        go straight to voicemail with no ring
the answer, though implicit, 's clear:
        No more, no more. Let silence sing.

The Binmen Are Coming

it's bin day
there is a low, distant rumble
coming from round the corner
somewhere, orange lights flash
seen reflected in windows
sounds of crushing hydraulics
and a warning chime

have I put the rubbish out
have we put the rubbish out
everything will be taken away

The Contents of a Desk Drawer

Highlighters in a wide range of colours

A plastic bag containing two dozen mysterious metal clips

A spent Oyster card

A fountain pen without a cartridge, long since unused

A bag of cartridges for said pen

A set of keys for a car now scrapped

Old diaries

Blu Tack

Elastic bands

A conjoined pair of postal stamps (1p and 2p)

Several dead watches

A passport

Cheque book stubs

A dried-up pen bearing the logo of a computer magazine
    that ceased publication 20 years ago

Staples (two sizes)

Fluff

Old front door keys

Half an inch of candle

Two treasury tags, green

Half a dozen paperclips, no two alike

A bottle of correction fluid

A pencil eraser into which the logo of a company I once ran was carved to form a stamp

A school "Vice Captain" badge, 1980s vintage

A bag of Swedish change

Four Scottish pound notes issued by three different banks

A not-quite-empty packet of Pritt Buddies (popularly known as "Pink Tack") from the late 70s, possibly early 80s: the price label reads "41p"

A Casio scientific calculator whose LED digits have probably not lit in 30 years

Lost youth

The States of Matter

The electric-plastic-manic world is gone.
There is just sky and sea and land –
  gas, liquid and solid –
  the three matter states,
  all suffused with life.

The air ripples with skylarks'
  voices of liquid . . . liquid . . . liquid;
at every step I am companioned by butterflies
  of summer orange and sun-dried brown;
waves interface with shingle
  and gently caress . . . caress . . . caress;
and from parched ground the purple and the yellow
  reach up in celebration of bloom.

The electric-plastic-manic world is gone.
There is just sky and sea and land –
  nothing else on this vital orb
  but you and me
  and all these lives.

Falling

A falling autumn dawn.

Anniversary eve, exploring Coigach:
Stac Pollaidh's jags in a cloud pewter shroud.

Tunnels of gold on the Mad Little Road;
forced to turn back by deepening floods.

Through the bleak beauty, kyle to kyle,
single-track-reaching the northmost of north.

Waking wet-eyed under luminous skies,
promising Caithness that we would return.

A falling autumn dawn.

Expectation

On Tuesday,
I knew it would rain,
and it came down like nails.
The forecast said gales:
I could just barely stand.
Red hail was predicted,
and it ruined the fruit.
They warned of tornadoes;
my car landed a mile off.
We all shrugged.

On Wednesday,
the weather was going to be awful,
the TV said.
So I took on extra work
and spent the day in the office,
toiling at my desk
and gazing out the window
at the rest of the world enjoying the last day of summer.
I felt monumentally hard done-by.

Aquarium

"Armitage Shanks",
it said on the toilet –
or rather "Arinitage Sharks",
as Harry thought it said.

He was still getting used to joined-up,
and the words were written
in a slightly unclear-to-him
script lettering.

"Sharks in the toilet?" he wondered,
excited and scared in equal measure.
(He guessed that "Arinitage" meant
something like "Warning".)

So he settled down gingerly,
did what he had to do, and left,
relieved but a little disappointed
that no sharks had put in an appearance –

not even a little one
like he had seen at the aquarium.
Not *really* dangerous,
but they could still bite

a bit –
Harry was sure of that.
What a tale that would've been.

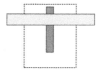

Xanthocryptus novozealandicus

Length: 12 mm; wingspan: 24 mm

A black-and-white ichneumon wasp native to New Zealand
that parasitises wood-boring beetles.

The Long Tail

(based on conversations with people with dementia, their families and carers)

To
begin in the middle –
which is, after all, where we are,
for if you are at the beginning you do not
know you are at the beginning, and if you are
at the end you do not know anything at all –
here we are. —— In any case, I can't recall when it
began, the long, slow tailing-off of your cometary path
of life. And though a tedious, drawn-out commentary is
not my intention, for now, the long tail fills my view. ——
When I rang today, they said: "He's very sleepy," as they
always seem to do these days. So they took the phone to you,
and I said "Hello," and you creaked "HELLO," so I asked you
how you were, and you answered as if in another present
"I'M ALL RIGHT," and then you fell asleep again and that was it.
So: "I'M ALL RIGHT." You're all right. By any reasonable
standard, you're not all right, but by the unreasonable
standard of this Thing, all right is what you are. What's left
is all right. Left as in remaining. Still present. A gift that
doesn't move. —— Doesn't move, like your hand, that
morning. That morning you rang me at seven and said: "I
THINK I'VE HAD A STROKE." That morning set us on a new
trail – a long tail – twisting between recovery and
decline. But that wasn't the beginning, I now
realise. —— A wasp sting deep in your brain (a
TIA – thanks in advance), and then another,
and again, drilling you with their long,
pointed tails, until at last their
nest (constructed
from

75

chewed fragments of your headwood, built to brood their tiny young) detonated. —— *Vespula vulgaris*, the common wasp. *Vespula*, vascular – they almost rhyme too much. The diagnosis was vascular dementia, caused by a major stroke. The paralysis down your left-hand side only lasted a week or so, fortunately, but the damage to your mind was permanent, and subsequently progressive. The holes blasted in your memory. The short-circuits. The personality twists. The callous destruction of everything that you were. —— Some stories start at the beginning. A stroke. A fall. A shocking change, like a rupture in reality. Some tales fade in diffusely, an unwanted broadcast bleeding through on the frequency, at first imperceptible, did I imagine that, that sounded like a different voice, a distant taxi firm, then again, then more frequent and insistent and undeniable, breaking up the programme so the music's gone, replaced by arguments and feedback and static. —— As a child, you met Marconi when he stayed with your family. You were a mother. You were a father. You were an artist. You were a musician. You were a baker. You were a biochemist. You worked with Marie Stopes. You were an engineer. You worked at Bletchley Park as a codebreaker. You trained at RADA. You marked O-level papers. You stacked shelves. You sang light opera. You were down the pits. You taught me to catch. You took me to see West Ham play. You travelled the world. You were loved by millions. You were loved by me. You cared for your parents in their old age. You photographed your family. And now, you're putting out cat litter for the birds to eat. Attempting to unlock the car with a chunk of lemon. Trying to fit both your fists in your mouth at the same time. —— It happened so gradually that at first I didn't notice it. You were so astute, you cleverly covered it over. But you couldn't cover what you couldn't control. The aggression. The anger. The frustration with yourself. —— Going back to zero. Having started there, and grown and lived and climbed all the ladders, it's like you're riding a snake all the way back down. Back down to zero. —— First signs. You were always jovial, kindhearted, there for everybody, big hugs and kisses – and this Thing robbed you of that. You stopped laughing. That was the first sign. —— You started saying strange things, like: "I SAW PAVAROTTI WHEN WE WERE OUT SHOPPING." In Swindon? On a bus? —— You had strategies for covering it up. Like if I asked for a cup of tea, you'd put the kettle on, and then there would be a pause and you'd say: "WELL, YOU KNOW HOW YOU LIKE IT. YOU COME AND MAKE IT." But I missed those early signs, until I asked you what the time was, and you said: "I DON'T KNOW, I CAN'T SEE THE CLOCK," but you could, I knew you could, you knew I knew you could, and that was an awful moment: the realisation, the panic on your face as you were looking at the clock and you just couldn't interpret it. —— The first thing I knew was when you told me. Such a clever man, you knew how to hide it. And you knew it wasn't just age, what was happening to your memory. You knew when to tell me. When to ask for help. —— We were playing chess, and you were winning, like you always used to. And then you made a mistake. Or rather, it wasn't you, it was the Thing inside you that made the mistake. Because you didn't make mistakes like that. So I took your queen, because what else could I do, and you just knocked all the pieces flying. Two hordes scattered to the winds. That wasn't like you at all: always such a calm and placid man. I'd never known you to get angry at anything, and now – and from then on – you were getting angry with things all the time. Or maybe you were getting angry with yourself. —— To begin in the middle, here we are.

—— We were in this art class, in a daycare centre, and you were just in tears. You'd always been a keen artist, but that day, at that moment, in that room, you suddenly realised you couldn't remember how to draw. You simply couldn't remember how to *do* it. And that was devastating. You just collapsed in sobs, and we had to help you out of the room. —— In hospital, after the stroke, you were hallucinating. Or rather, I see in retrospect, you were dreaming. No, you're still in the same hospital. Yes, really. No, they didn't take you to London. Was it that you were unused to being able to remember your dreams? Or was it that you were unable to distinguish between dreams and reality? —— It was the question that sideswiped me. "WHAT'S THE MATTER WITH THAT FRONT DOOR?" "Pardon, what?" "THE LOCK'S ALL DETACHED FROM IT." "What do you mean, Dad?" "WELL, IT'S SORT OF FLOATING ABOUT IN SPACE." And then, after that, you didn't seem to be the same person. —— You were convinced they were trying to poison you. You became very suspicious, accusatory – and preoccupied with the toilet: you would flush everything you could get hold of down the toilet. And then there were the violent rages. You would hit him. Harm him. And he just took it. Eventually we got you to the doctor, and when the doctor told you: "You have Alzheimer's," you got up and punched him on the nose. Blood everywhere. —— To middle in the middle, we are. —— The human brain is the strangest and most wonderful object in the universe, three pounds of wet, grey extraordinariness. And even when it's been badly degraded by this horrible Thing, it can still find something amusing. The humour is still there, which I suppose is reassuring. But it's also heart-wrenching. If I can make you laugh, I see you again. And sometimes your mum. I see her. —— If you were being cantankerous, I'd give you a packet of Everton Mints, or put some Doris Day on, and that would keep you happy. —— The family didn't believe that you had dementia. I mean, you were living with us, and I saw what you were like every day, but they lived a long way away and they would visit once every six weeks or something. And they would say: "I don't know why you keep saying Dad has dementia. He hasn't got dementia. I can sit there and have a perfectly normal conversation with him." But they were just getting these tiny, normal snapshots, not what you were really like. So they didn't believe me. And after that they wouldn't speak to me. Not until after the funeral. They just thought I was being horrible about you. But why would I make it up? —— When we didn't know what else to do to engage you, we would put *Mr Bean* on the TV, and you would sit there and just *laugh*. When you were younger, you'd have been going: "What is that silly man doing?", but now he was doing these stupid things and you thought it was hysterical. —— I turned up one evening and you'd got all the torches in bits on the kitchen table. I asked you why you'd taken them apart, and you said: "I WAS JUST CHECKING THEY WORK." —— You stopped answering questions. "OH, I DON'T KNOW," you would say, giving up halfway through a sentence. "I DON'T KNOW." Your personality didn't change as the dementia progressed. You just sort of lost your personality: the edges became a bit more woolly and you gradually sort of faded away, like an old tape recording. "I DON'T KNOW." —— You started to get obsessed with tyre pressures. Every two hours, you'd be going out to the car to check the tyres. —— You started to question where you were. "IS THIS HOME?" In your mind, one moment you were in your childhood home and then suddenly you were somewhere else you didn't recognise. —— We are in the middle of the muddle. —— You were happy in your little world. A dream to look after, as long as you had your knitting and your feather duster. —— And now you don't recognise your wife, your husband, your child, your home, yourself. "WHO ARE YOU?" you ask. —— You took the locks off all the doors. And obsessed with emptying the fridge, you were. Hated having food in the fridge, so you'd throw it out into the garden. —— People don't invite us out anymore. They don't realise that you can still hold a normal conversation. They think the diagnosis means you've gone doolally, but that's not it at all: all your thought processes are still there, they just take longer. It's like an old computer: however slow it is, and however frustrating it is to watch the hourglass on the screen, shouting won't help. I just have to be patient. I know you'll get there. You forget words, and you have to find alternatives. Sometimes the alternatives make sense, and sometimes they don't. We still laugh, we still dream, we still love, even though you lose words. So we hold the-things-on-the-ends-of-our-arms, and when there's something you want to tell me and you hit a roadblock, you have to circum—, er, something, go round the, er, bushes, while you're slowly trying to make your point. I don't mind waiting. —— Remembering when you'd just had the diagnosis. They had done scans and shown you the damage. What was it you said to me? "I'M AMAZED I'M STILL HERE." —— One day you were talking with great lucidity about an airshow you'd gone to. You described all the planes, all the people you met, all the detail. "THE RED ARROWS DID A FLY PAST" – and then the façade slipped – "AND THEY WERE SO LOW, I GOT CAUGHT ON THE UNDERCARRIAGE OF ONE OF THE PLANES AND WAS CARRIED UP INTO THE SKY." —— Some days, one wouldn't know anything was wrong. Other days, I can't get a word out of you. A shell, a hollow husk. And it's hard not to wonder if this is me in twenty-odd years. Or less. —— You were always so active and interested. You'd always ask: "WHAT CAN I DO TO HELP?" So I'd ask you to peel the carrots, and you would get on with that, but you would have that carrot peeled right down to a point – like an offensive weapon. You'd start peeling it, and you wouldn't think: "I've got all the peel off" and move on to the next one, you'd just carry on paring that one carrot. And while you were peeling, you'd be talking, and gesturing, holding the knife, and it wasn't a safe place to be. But you just wanted to help. —— Sometimes it's like you're standing in fog and you don't know where you are. It's hard to believe you were once such a dignified woman. I can see in your eyes that you're trying to understand what I'm saying – staring intently at me as your brain battles to make the right connections – but you get so frustrated. The dignity has been stripped from you. This Thing is ruthless, degrading. —— We are in the middle middle. —— I remember Dad trying to cover for you when you started to drink heavily. That happens, doesn't it? The one without dementia covers for the one with. Of course, you had no notion of how much brandy you were copiously downing. And he was trying to drink it quicker than you so it would all be gone and you couldn't have any. That worked for a while, until he got drunk and passed out. —— To begin with, it was just forgetfulness, and I could cope with that, but when it reached the stage where there was no recognition *it changed me.* I stopped being a wife, and started being a carer, because that was the only way, mentally, that I could deal with it. Once I'd made that transition, it made things a bit easier: in my mind, I'd taken away my husband and replaced him with a person that needed me. I emotionally detached myself to protect myself. Sometimes I look back and I think, how selfish was that? Because when you would ask me: "WHEN'S MY WIFE COMING HOME?", instead of responding by saying: "But I am your wife," I'd say: "Well, I don't really know, but will I do for now?" Should I have fought more to make you recognise me? It seemed like such a hard battle that I'd never win. —— I lost you long before you'd gone. —— In the care home, I'd go and visit, and sometimes I'd look at you and think you were dead, and other times you'd be sitting up cheerfully and chatting with me and not have a clue who I was. The last time you stayed with us, you didn't really know who we were, and I found that horrible. It must have been horrible for you. But you were very easily amused. You would knit, but you'd have no idea what you were making. And considering how brilliant you'd been at that kind of thing, your knitting now was full of holes and dropped stitches and stuff. And because I didn't have very much wool, when you went to bed in the evening I'd unravel it all, like Penelope, and then the next day you'd start again and happily knit away with the same wool, knitting the holes in your mind and dropping stitches like memories. —— Sometimes it's been said that dementia reveals the true person, or it magnifies faults, but I don't believe that. The way that Alzheimer's breaks connections and makes new connections that don't make any sense – that can have any effect at all. It can easily change personalities. He was always very chatty and friendly and calm and kind, which makes it all the more horrible when dementia turns someone like that into an angry person. I knew an old lady who was ever so sweet until she got dementia; she was asked to leave her warden-controlled accommodation when she took an axe to the wardrobe and smashed it up. Then she went for a walk, waded into the middle of the river and refused to come out. Disturbs the residents, that kind of thing. —— You're always eating. I wake at 3 a.m., see the hall lights on, get up and find you in the kitchen eating some strange breakfast you've composed. And then the same thing happens again at six. During the day, you're normally tramping around, moving things from room to room. But if it all goes quiet, I'll know you're in the kitchen eating something - probably from the fruit bowl or the biscuit barrel. We have to keep the fruit bowl topped up, otherwise you'll polish off all the biscuits. —— You would escape from respite care: the police would find you wandering the streets, stealing ice creams off children, leaving a trail of destruction. But by then, you weren't talking. Didn't speak a word for the last fifteen years of your life. I would hold your hand and talk and tell you things, but there would be no response at all. —— "INEXPERIENCED AS I AM IN MORE THAN NOTHING," you said. "IT'S QUITE FUNNY, REALLY," you said, four times in a row. "PLEASE GET ME OW," you said, over and over again. Nonsense as these were, I'd settle for them instead of the silence there is now. —— There was the bit when you'd keep asking after your parents, parents who'd been gone decades. Or the dog. You were always asking where the dog was. And every time you found out your mum was dead, or that the dog had passed away, you felt the loss afresh, and in the end I just had to stop telling you, to stop distressing you, so I'd change the subject or evade the question. And I felt so guilty, like I was manipulating you, like I was fabricating a wall of lies, but I had to live in your world, where time had disconnected, nothing was linear, everything you'd ever done was happening now, apart from the things you couldn't remember, which was almost everything. Left with particles of memory, floating about in space. Like the comet's tail. —— You were always the person everyone went

83

to for advice. Whatever it was, whoever it was asking, you would be so kind. —— We need to talk. The problem is, you can't talk any more. —— Yesterday, you were having such a "good day" they called me so we could talk on the phone. All smiles and playing Scrabble, they said. But that's not what I got. You laid down plenty of words, true, but zero points for comprehension. Instead there was bewilderment; frustration; pain. Probably the first time I've heard you say anything other than single words in months. I'm glad the care assistant enjoyed your company. But now   it's the small hours. I've woken from a dream   in which you make sense and you understand and we can talk and you're fine for one day and we rejoice and make the most of it, knowing that it won't last, and it doesn't, because it was a dream, and here I am, and there you are. It is mid April. A late frost has browned the blooms of next door's magnolia, and soon the ground beneath the tree will be thick with loss. —— At night, if I suddenly make a noise, I tell myself: "Quiet, or you'll wake him." Then it hits me that you're not there. Like you're dead. But yours is a living death. —— There were days, well, moments, when you still had a spark. You always did like the word "thixotropic". It reminded you of your food science experiments. Rheology. "What's the opposite of thixotropic?" I asked. "THINOTROPIC," you said, with a grin and a twinkle. —— By steps, you lost your English, reverted to Greek, your mother tongue. That caused problems at the care home. Every day, I'd get a phone call: could I talk to you, find out what you're trying to say, translate. —— I look back now with fondness, but at the time I could have climbed the walls sometimes. ——

"PLEASE CAN YOU PUT MLNZMMLNMM." "Come again?"
"PLEASE CAN YOU PUT MLNZMLN FOOD." "Something about
food?" "YES."

"You want to eat something?" "YES."
"What do you want to eat?" "ANYTHING THAT MOVES."
——

We muddle of the
  middle. This monster that's twisted your melon, smashed
and withered your walnut, minced your prime fillet steak.
—— "I'VE GOT SOME FROZEN IN THE FISH," you said, looking in

the oven and
wondering why it wasn't cold. —— I took you to visit Dad in
hospital. While we were there, the nurse had to attend to
him, so we left

    the room, and when we came back
        five minutes later you said: "WHERE IS HE, THEN?"
    "He's there in the bed, Mum." "THAT'S NOT HIM, THAT'S
AN OLD MAN." "How old is Dad, do you think?" "HE'S IN HIS
40S." So you'd lost 40 years in five minutes. After
Dad died, we told you and
you said: "OH, I WONDERED WHAT HAD
                        HAPPENED TO HIM." Your own
husband, but you didn't miss him. You didn't really know
who he was any more. ——

"PUT ME TO BED. PUT ME TO BED. PUT ME TO BED. PUT ME TO BED.
PLEASE PUT ME TO BED." "You *are* in bed." "*PLEASE PUT ME TO*

BED. PLEASE PUT ME TO BED. " ——
Now we are
      separate bones, no more rattling together.
    Sort of floating about   in space.

          Wearing half a tie. Thixotropic and calm.
     Inexperienced as I

am in more than nothing. In the   middle. The long tail.
I'm here. I'm still
                here,   in

      the comet's tail. It's hard
     to see out, past the dust and glowing gas.
Once in a while, I get a glimpse
  of the   else,

          the rest, the non-tail.   A moment
   of clarity. And then
the white noise-fog returns. Put
the lemon in the

     the place.

Put it.
  No, the lem

   .   What can I help?
    What *can?*   In the

muddle, I catch a wasp. Nothing is

linear, everything   disconnects,   every
sense short-   circuits, dreaming   in
        the   light, in the

                                dark light, *pour-*

                                                                    quoi,
        it's quite funny really, funnyreal, funereal,
unravelling the

                        wall, knitting   memories from
        scattered
                    mints, a   diagnosis
                                            of three-day

weeks, c   limb   ing   up to
        zero, stucks in

                    angry, flushing all the
        food downup

                                    the fridger and find
        me sleep onthe   lawn

                                                covered   in
        orangepeelandslugss.

All the words.

None of the words.

And   all be

cause

the

Thing ate

you. And the shape of

this

outrage?

A long

tail.

Dicopomorpha echmepterygis

Length: 186 μm

With an average length of less than 0.2 mm,
males of this wasp species are the smallest known insects.
They are blind and have no wings.

sleep-starved,
I yawn;
the day starts
despite me

dead wasp
on windowsill;
would sting me
if it could

with every step
sparks fly off the grass –
    sun on frost

        vapour rising:
            the river's warm breath escapes
            into the cool dawn

after the showers,
      the sun shines green oaks vivid
      and zinc poplars glint

            above the river,
            a galaxy of midges –
                whirling traffic

cherry tree
just one branch in blossom
    late November

you say there are no hard feelings
but you're wrong:
all feelings are difficult

                    every cloud
                    looks like you
                    today;
                    how come

                                        every time
                                        we connect,
                                        I fear
                                        it's the last

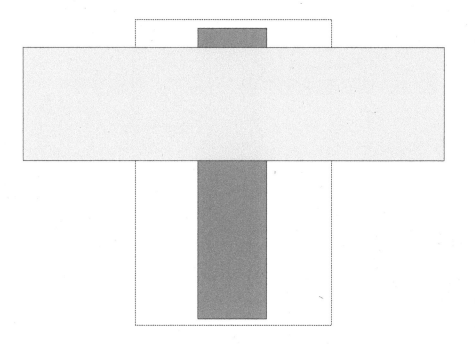

Megascolia procer

Length: 77 mm; wingspan: 116 mm

The giant scoliid wasp, native to Java and Sumatra.
It has iridescent wings, which are absolutely entrancing
if you can stand to hang around long enough.

Windfalls

The tired old apple tree faded
two years ago, the branches
now barkless and fruitless.

I will just one more speckled orb
to form on your aged limbs;
the slim hope of a glimmer

of life keeps me going,
clinging to trees' and parents'
wisdom long after the sap's dried.

Autumn is coming;
what will the wasps do
without the windfall feast?

Never Gelati

I have tasted many memorable ice creams
in locations both ugly and picturesque,
but what of it?
Why would you want to hear about *them*?
"Oh, I had the most divine camel's milk ice cream,"
I might begin to recount,
and already you would have switched off
long before I started to describe the exotic flavour
    combination concerned,
because that's just bragging,
and who wants to hear that?

No, the strongest memories
and the ones I hope you might spare a moment for
are the ice creams I never got to try –
my never gelati, if you will.

September 2012, in Calvi, Corsica:
a tiny backstreet room selling one thing only –
limoncello gelato.
It was our last day there,
and that morning I was much reduced in strength
by stomach cramps.
I simply couldn't.
We never went back,
but still I recall the simple chalk-on-blackboard sign outside
and that never gelato.

September 2017, in Rome:
on our last morning,

en route to the airport,
we made a special detour to a highly recommended
    gelateria
in expectation of extraordinary tastes.
But alas,
despite the protestations of the sign on the door
that they opened at eleven,
here we were at quarter past
and there was no sign of life.
After loitering a few minutes,
we moved on, a plane to catch,
leaving behind my fig and walnut never gelato.

October 2020, in Dymchurch, Kent:
another sunny autumn day
requiring frozen churned refreshment:
a little shop selling their own freshly made gelato,
and the flavour on the board that made me gasp:
Turkish delight – quince and rose.
So why, this time, would this be a never gelato?
Just 30 seconds before,
at the ice cream kiosk next door,
we had just bought a cone each of that day's special:
amaretto and cherry bakewell flavour.
It was very good indeed.
But I can't help wondering what the other one would have
    been like.
And I can't imagine ever seeing
Turkish delight – quince and rose gelato
on sale again.

Three never gelati.

Appropriate Verse Form

I was translating this Norwegian government report, as you do – well, I do, pays the bills and that – and it was all about what needs to be done to encourage and protect pollinating insects. We all know about the bees being in decline and the potential for "cascading effects on food webs" (as it says here), but this was quite a positive document about safeguarding biodiversity, the success of various initiatives and "proactive measures going forward".

And then it made reference to some recent German research that stopped me translating mid sentence.

This study showed a decrease in flying insect biomass over 27 years (from 1989 to 2016) of *more than 75 per cent.*

The shocking thing about it is that that's not the shocking thing about it.

The shocking thing about it is that the research wasn't done in urban areas, or farmland, but in *nature reserves.*

So basically, if we assume that this is a trend not just in German nature reserves but generally – at least, in this part of the world – that would mean that (as an exceedingly rough approximation) three-quarters of all the flying insects have disappeared since I left school. Yes, that means the bees. Yes, the butterflies too. And the wasps, the moths, the flying beetles, the greenbottles, the midges, the mozzies, the hornets, the hoverflies, the crickets, the dragonflies – presumably even the daddy-long-legs.

That decline must be at least partly my fault. My net effect on the planet's ecosystem has been negative.

And so to commemorate this realisation I decided to write a limerick. To subvert the medium. To use what is normally a humorous verse form to point up a horrifying truth. And this is what I came up with:

There once was a study in Germany
Conducted to find out just how many
Flying insects aloft are;
It turns out that there are far
Fewer than in the past, and much less honey.

Does that work? I don't know really. I'd hoped it would make a powerful point, but now I'm worrying that it just makes a serious and tragic subject sound a bit silly.

On the other hand, that 75 per cent decline in insect numbers will certainly stick in the mind now.

Nothing*

---

* Except everything.

Ox Drove
(for Terry and Nicky)

To follow this track,
as drovers and pilgrims have done
    since Domesday alike,
is to amble the æons:
a wide valley view,
scarcely changed for generations
    of travellers and trees,
rewards and refreshes
the post Space Age eye.

We walk, untroubled by traffic
save for insect attention:
bees en route from bramble to bramble;
occasional air-shuffling pockets
    of midge-crammed anger;
and then – *butterfly* –
a Painted Lady, weary and worn
    from her flight from the Med,
more pastel-paint than bright now
but still alive, aloft –
with every wingbeat
the sensation is that of
millennia collapsing.

Notebook

Turning the page,
I wait for the words to come
but all I can see
is the past
in faint mirror image
through the paper –
always with us
until we replace the book.

WASP DISENTANGLEMENT FOR BEGINNERS

Morning Walks Two

Six minutes, front door to field gate.
The hedgerows' naked oaks are alive with birds.
A mile away, a yaffle twangs a six-inch ruler on a desk.

I stop to talk to a chap walking his dogs.
He explains all this is going: six hundred houses.
After twenty minutes, he apologises for ranting.

A skylark sings.

Cœur

(compiled entirely from words found in a
glossary of nuclear energy)

highly enriched for natural abundance
with an elastic emulsion to stretch age,
tissue equivalent epithermal cascade
and well-moderated fertile fraction

shimming reactivity feed-back:
the minimum critical infinite slab
of moderate void upscattering method
and gray cut curie buckling

virgin neutron vitrification;
phantom tolerance of burst slug
down by the fission spike;
cold shutdown on cold shutdown

the fail-safe chop of turn-around time,
parasitic flux density and thimble count;
rabbit shuttle subcooled boiling –
an exemption from the nozzle process

out to the hot lead labyrinth,
in scintillating sun-burst skyshine,
supercritical decay on xenon override
and lethal tritium glove box dummy

isodose lethargy cake:
the macroscopic crud blanket
of dollar event albedo containment,
without exclusion, without tail, without end

Porthluney

I've been here before.
Not in a past-life sense
but in a this-life sense:
I've been here with you,
I've been here without you,
I've been here with friends,
I've been here with family
and God willing
I'll come back here again with you one day;
because every time,
this place brings calm,
and I love sharing that with you.

Hedychrum rutilans

Length: 7 mm; wingspan: 11.4 mm

A species of cuckoo wasp found in continental Europe.
The female is metallic green-and-red,
like an imagined jewel.

Note: The first seven parts of Sanity Sparrows appeared in the pamphlet On Wings. *With the additional parts collected here, the sequence is now complete.*

Sanity Sparrows

I.

I feel rubbish.
I feel rubbish.
I feel rubbish.
I feel rubbish.

I step outside the front door,
stop,
and listen. A score of sparrows
in next door's hedge
are loudly expressing their joy
at existence.

I feel lighter.
I feel calmer.
Even back inside the house, door closed,
I can still hear the sparrows' chatter,
a precious reminder
of that reassurance.

II.

Exuberantly,
the sparrows are playing tag
in the trees next door.

III.

A lone blackbird,
sharp in dark suit
and loud orange beak,
gatecrashes the sparrows' tree party.

After an uneasy stand-off,
a nearby sound startles all the attendees
and together they retreat
into the hidey-hedge,
united in dense safety and truce.

IV.

First morning of national lockdown.
I watch the birds out there,
my sanity sparrows.
Through them, I enjoy vicarious freedom,
their close social interaction.
Through them, I fly.

V.

Although there is bright sunshine,
the wind is cruel and cold.

Although they could be flying,
the sparrows hunker in the hedge.

Although I could take my daily walk,
I too am sheltering in warmth.

VI.

Another tantalisingly bright morning.
A distant chiming bell counts seven
as I sit on the front doorstep,
unable to take an early walk
because that would mean no walk together later.

There are five sparrows on my neighbours' roof,
a gathering legal by dint of species.
One of them was thrown in for free;
but of course they are all free,
and the whirr of their wingbeats
as they commute between hedge and eaves
is the sound of freedom.

VII.

A couple of months into This Thing,
the trees of the hedge are now in leaf
and the sparrows' noisy perches are largely hidden.
But I can still hear them,
my companions of cheer.

There's a patch of grit at the side of the road,
a spot untouched by wheel or shoe
where fine material collects.
The sparrows use it as a dust bath,
taking turns to soothe their irritations.

Watching them, I find my face to be aching.

VIII.

sparrow voices always there
day on hour
week on day
month on week
I hear your constancy from where I lie troubled

what are you
winged sparks
morsels of life
symbolic presences
a collective consciousness
particles in constant flux
bound by interaction
just as we are
a reminder of cohesive strength
and mutual support

when I ache to my feathertips from the effort of staying aloft
maybe I should chirp more
roost more
flock more
be more sparrow

IX.

Out by the drop kerb,
the sparrows are pecking
at atoms of food.

In the half-dozen group,
sometimes one will turn on another,
taking offence at some slight or encroachment.
The argument flashes up like powder in a pan,
the birds scatter, reassemble,
and all is peace once more.

O that human squabbles
had a half-life so short,
fading into forgotten
within a half-dozen seconds.

X.

They've gone.
This morning,
there are no sparrows to be perceived.

But their absence –
their not-being –
is louder than the song of their presence.

A resounding
negative space
that chimes with truth and beauty.

XI.

I sit at my desk,
work undone.
My eyes defocus
until the print on the page
is just a grey fog.

Outside,
the sparrows get on with their morning jobs
in easy chatter.

Words coalesce on the page before me:
"All is well.
All is well.
All is well.
All is well."

The Wasps of Memory

Circa 1989:
a visit to my paternal grandmother,
a formidable late-Victorian lady
whom Wodehouse would have enjoyed describing.

We were accompanying her
on a brief constitutional near her Sussex home
when my father and I noticed and remarked upon
the sight of two wasps on the pavement,
apparently engaged in a brutal fight to the death.

"Probably just having sex," harrumphed Granny,
and shuffled on.

Me and Dad just looked at each other in astonishment
that such a cast-iron prude as our aged r.
(who could not even bring herself to utter the word
    "bottom",
yet swore in German – a relic of Swiss finishing school)
would have said such a thing.

And she was wrong.
That's not how they mate,
as far as I can tell.
I mean, I'm not an expert on wasps or anything.

Acknowledgements

I wish to thank all those who kindly and anonymously gave their time and shared their experiences of dementia in all its forms. Your generous help made The Long Tail possible.

Tusen takk to Reidar and Rune for Norwegian advice and feedback.

Love and thanks to Steph for patience and inspiration.

And to Rita: Thanks for the wasp.

Index

Note: Untitled poems are listed by their first line or lines.

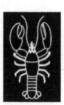

This is Leon.
Leon appreciates wasps for their utility.
But then, as a lobster living underwater,
he's never been stung by one.